30 Weeks to Awesome.

Your Step-by-Step Guide to Building Healthy Habits

Elizabeth J. Smith

DISCLAIMER

The content of this book is for general informational purposes only. It is
not meant to be used, nor should it be used, to diagnose or treat any
medical condition or to replace the services of your physician or other
healthcare provider. The advice and strategies contained in the book may
not be suitable for all readers. Please consult your healthcare provider for
any questions that you may have about your own medical situation. Neither
the author, publisher, IIN nor any of their employees or representatives
guarantees the accuracy of information in this book or its usefulness to a
particular reader, nor are they responsible for any damage or negative
consequence that may result from any treatment, action taken, or inaction
by any person reading or following the information in this book.

In other words…please do not do anything stupid. I do not know your
particular situation. Use your common sense and consult your physician,
who understands your personal situation, at all times.

Institute of Integrative Nutrition and IIN are trademarks of Integrative
Nutrition, Inc.

~ In love, and peace, and health

Liz

CONTENTS

ACKNOWLEDGMENTS

This journey started in 2016 during a health coaching program called Swim, Bike, Fuel, designed and led by Meredith Vieccelli and Meredith Atwood. The program no longer exists, but both women continue their work improving the lives of other people. I thank them deeply for that course. Shortly thereafter, I enrolled at the Institute for Integrative Nutrition (IIN). IIN is truly creating a powerful ripple effect that has touched the lives of thousands, and probably millions of people. It was at IIN that I deepened my understanding of health in a more holistic way, and the curriculum inspired me to continue to spread that knowledge using 1:1 coaching and other resources such as this book.

This book could not have been created without the support of my husband, Quinn. He supported my crazy ideas and showed tremendous patience as I searched for and began to create a career and life I love. As a new and self-published author, I thought long and hard about whether to invest in the help of others. I am so glad that I did: this book is so, so much better thanks to the help of my editor, Lera O'Sullivan, because of the cover design and publishing consultation by Anita Roche, and the back cover photography by Patrick Barry. Thanks also to the various friends and to my Aunt Patricia, who looked at portions of the book and provided suggestions. Thanks especially to Alasen Zarndt and Kari Fenske for pre-reading the book and sharing their thoughts. It takes a community to create a book and to put it out in the world. Thank you, community: to those mentioned and those I may have missed.

WELCOME To your 30-week wellness journal!

Congratulations on taking this huge step towards improving your health! I am guessing that you feel as though work, while hopefully satisfying, has taken over your life. You may have spent years prioritizing your career over your personal life, while your health has slowly deteriorated. That is going to change in the next 30 weeks. You will learn how to create health without making it a second career. You will put the 'life' back into your work life balance. By making small changes each day over the next 30 weeks, you will start on a journey that will make you happier and more productive all around: at work, in your relationships, and at home.

Each week will include a new lesson along with an action item. Some actions will be habits that you can incorporate each day in the week. Sometimes it may take a full week to implement the action item (and sometimes it may even carry over into other weeks). Following each lesson are pages to record your thoughts and progress each day.

I will provide information and action steps, but the transformation is up to you. Plan to spend 3-10 minutes per day on the action item, and another two minutes to keep track of your progress by recording your thoughts on your new habits and using the checklists on each page. The checklists will build each week as a quick reminder of the habits you are building.

If you are traveling or feeling stuck and ready to stop working through this book, turn to the two bonus sections at the end for guidance.

Remember, this is the start of a journey, not the end. Have fun, have compassion for yourself and your pace of change, and let's get started!

Sincerely,
Liz Smith, Integrative Nutrition Health Coach

LESSON RECAP
Each week the highlights of the weekly lesson will be described here.

ACTION ITEM You will receive a small action item each week for the next 30 weeks. It will be highlighted for you here.

HEALTHY HABIT CHECKLIST
The checklist will remind you of topics already covered in preceding weeks. You can mark off each day, or go through the checklist each week to see what you have accomplished. This is a reminder. It does not mean you need to keep up with everything every week.

Journal Pages Format
Take a minute or two each day to check in with yourself about the weekly action item, your progress on goals you continue to work on from prior weeks, as well as how you are feeling, other thoughts, etc. You can also record your reasoning if you did not follow through on something. This will allow you to revisit your decisions to determine if you have a pattern of making specific excuses to avoid certain things.

Monday: _____
_____
_____
_____
_____

Tuesday: _____
_____
_____
_____

Wednesday:_____
_____
_____
_____
_____

WEEK ONE

WHERE ARE YOU NOW?

"If you cannot measure it, you cannot manage it."
~ Lord Kelvin

Before you start to focus on change, get clear on where you are currently. When our habits change, it is easy to forget where we were in the past because the new habit becomes so strong. This is particularly true when making small changes that do not feel difficult, but will transform your life over time.

To mark this period as you begin your health transformation, do the following three things this week. These will focus on different aspects of your life to get your snapshot.

1. Fill out the circle of life on the following page. Place a dot in the wedge for each category to indicate your level of satisfaction in that area. The center of the circle indicates zero satisfaction in that area; the outer edge indicates complete satisfaction in that area. Satisfaction means you do not feel there is room for improvement at this time in your life. Focus only on how you feel at this time. For example, education may not play a big role in your life right now, but if you are completely satisfied and do not wish to increase its role at this time, then you would put your dot near the outer edge of the circle. When you are done, connect the dots.

2. Take your physical measurements. Even if you do not want to lose weight your body may transform in the next thirty weeks – you will not know if you don't get your starting point. Use a flexible tape measure and record measurements on the opposite page.

3. Record the reasons you are committed to transforming your health in the next thirty weeks. What do you hope to get out of it?

Date: _____

1.

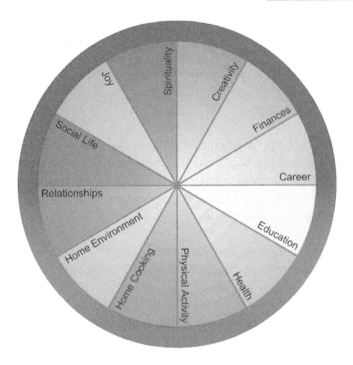

2.

	Start date_____	End Date _____
Neck		
Upper arm, widest part		
Bust – just under armpits		
Chest – directly under breast line		
Waist – smallest part of waist line		
Stomach – largest part of waistline		
Hips – largest area around your butt		
Upper thigh in widest area		

4

3.

I am choosing to spend 30 weeks building habits that will improve my

health because: _____

_____

_____

_____

I want to improve my health because it will allow me to: _____

_____

_____

_____

I can't wait to feel: _____

_____

I acknowledge that my biggest barriers will be: _____

_____

_____

_____

These are the people who will support me: _____

_____

WEEK ONE

Monday: _____
_____
_____
_____
_____

LESSON RECAP
In this first week,
take time to
recognize and
measure where
you are now.

Tuesday: _____
_____
_____
_____
_____

ACTION ITEMS
This week:
1) track your
current
satisfaction with
different areas of
your life,
2) measure
yourself physically,
3) reflect on why
you want to
transform your
health and why
you are committed
to this journal.

Wednesday:_____
_____
_____
_____
_____

Thursday: _____
_____
_____
_____
_____

HEALTHY HABIT CHECKLIST
□ Remember where you started & why

Friday: _____

_____

_____

_____

_____

Saturday:_____

_____

_____

_____

_____

Sunday:_____

_____

_____

_____

_____

Weekly Summary: _____

_____

_____

_____

_____

_____

_____

_____

_____

WEEK TWO

"If you can imagine it, you can achieve it."
~William Arthur Ward

Last week you got clear on where you are now, why you want to transform your health, and why you are committed to this journal. This week, the focus is to clarify where you are going. You will dive deeper and get more in-depth on your goals for the next 30 days, 90 days, and 210 days (the completion of this 30-week program).

The goals you set can be small or huge, but they should be written in such a way that you will know when you have achieved them. Your goals should be health-related, but health can be viewed very broadly. The circle of life that you completed last week touched on many aspects of life, all of which are connected to your health. Write out one to three goals for each time period.

If you are struggling, look back at your notes from last week. What brought you to this program and what do you want out of it? How can you rewrite those motivations into measurable goals? Look back over the circle of life. Where are you low, and what's one thing you can do to boost your satisfaction in that area of your life? If you want to eat better, how would that look? Perhaps eating at home at least 3 nights a week? Or eating 5 servings of vegetables a day? Do you want to start moving more? How about starting with 15 minutes of activity per week? Notice that all these examples put you in control. Choose goals, at least for the short-term, that feel ridiculously easy. Some progress is better than none.

You may be thinking: isn't this program to teach me what to do for my health? Yes, to an extent, but you already know right now some things you can do to improve your health. Here is your chance to get clear on what's most important. If you do not yet have all your goals filled out, revisit these pages throughout this program as you learn about health and identify areas in which you can improve, and ways to do it.

30 Days

    1. _____

    _____

    2. _____

    _____

    3. _____

    _____

90 Days

    1. _____

    _____

    2. _____

    _____

    3. _____

    _____

210 Days

    1. _____

    _____

    2. _____

    _____

    3. _____

    _____

WEEK TWO

LESSON RECAP
This week is about getting more specific on your goals moving forward and what you would like to achieve in 30 days, 90 days, and 210 days.

ACTION ITEMS
Write down your health-related goals, which can pertain to nearly everything in your life. Make sure they are specific and measurable so that you will know you have achieved them. Write at least one goal for each time period - 30 days, 90 days, and 210 days. Take the entire week to think about your upcoming goals.

Monday: _____

_____

_____

_____

_____

Tuesday: _____

_____

_____

_____

Wednesday:_____

_____

_____

_____

_____

Thursday: _____

_____

_____

_____

WEEK TWO

HEALTHY HABIT CHECKLIST
☐ Remember where you started & why
☐ Remember your goals

Friday: _____

_____
_____
_____
_____
_____

Saturday:_____

_____
_____
_____
_____

Sunday:_____

_____
_____
_____
_____

Weekly Summary: _____

_____
_____
_____
_____
_____
_____
_____

WEEK THREE

WATER

"Take care of your body. It's the only place you have to live."
~Jim Rohn

Your body needs water to function optimally. Most of us are not getting enough. When you are dehydrated, your body does not burn fat effectively because it is perceiving dehydration as a state of stress.

Staying hydrated may also help reduce cravings for sugar and other foods, improve skin health, reduce headaches, increase energy, and decrease muscle aches.

The amount needed depends on a variety of factors, but the general rule of thumb is to consume half of your body weight in ounces. Therefore, if you weigh 200 pounds, you should drink 100 ounces of water per day.

Spend the first three days this week monitoring how much water you currently consume. Don't make changes yet: instead figure out an accurate baseline.

If your baseline is less than half your weight in ounces, start adding water each day for the rest of the week. Start with an extra glass, about 8 ounces. Continue adding slowly until you reach your goal of half your weight in ounces. Use this journal to record how you feel. Once you hit the target of half your bodyweight in ounces, if you are feeling great then try to stick with it. You may not need quite that much, or you may need more. When you exercise you will need more than when you do not exercise. Trust your body as your guide based on when you are feeling your best. You may not think dehydration is affecting you, but you will not know until you experience life hydrated.

Take sips throughout the day, rather than consuming large amounts at any one time or only drinking with meals. When calculating your water consumption, only include water and herbal teas.

Monday: _____

_____

_____

_____

_____

LESSON RECAP
Water is important for our bodies to function optimally. Dehydration could be holding you back from feeling your best, and what is an easier and cheaper way to improve health than to drink water?

Tuesday: _____

_____

_____

_____

_____

ACTION ITEM
Starting this week, pay attention to how much water you consume daily and then start drinking more. Drink sips slowly throughout the day rather than all at once.

Wednesday:_____

_____

_____

_____

_____

Thursday: _____

_____

_____

_____

Don't like the taste of water? You can experiment with adding natural whole-food flavorings such as lemon or lime juice (or slices), orange slices, cucumber, mint leaves, or a dash of apple cider vinegar (also good for digestion).

HEALTHY HABIT CHECKLIST
□ Remember where you started & why
□ Remember your goals
□ Drink water

Friday: _____

_____

_____

_____

_____

Saturday:_____

_____

_____

_____

_____

Sunday:_____

_____

_____

_____

_____

Weekly Summary: _____

_____

_____

_____

_____

_____

_____

_____

WEEK FOUR

ADD IN TO CROWD OUT

"The habits that took years to build do not take a day to change."
~Susan Powter

This program is about making small changes that add up over time. It is about long-lasting habit change, not the kind of quick fix or drastic change that will inevitably have you returning back to your 'normal' habits before you even realize that it happened.

One of the concepts that can help you make these changes is to focus on what you are adding to your lifestyle, rather than to focus on removing the 'bad' stuff, which can make you feel as though you are missing out on something. For example, you can focus on eating more vegetables rather than restricting your food intake by volume.

As you add in the good, it will crowd out the bad. More importantly, by thinking about what to add and not what to take away, the change will feel like one of abundance, not restriction. Focus on what you choose to eat because of how it makes you feel, not based on what you think is bad for you. If you want to eat something that you consider unhealthy, then do so. Be aware of what you are eating and enjoy it rather than feeling guilty or bad about wanting to eat it. If you realize that the 'bad' food makes you want to take a nap, take note. Similarly, if you have a breakfast that keeps you satisfied, focused, and energized until lunch, notice that feeling.

Later in this program we will cover the concept of the 80/20 rule, or the idea that we can and should eat foods that we enjoy – these might not be the perfect foods but they may be accompanied by an emotional connection or may feed us in other ways such as memories or social connection.

LESSON RECAP
As we get into food and habit change throughout this program, focus on an abundance mindset of adding good, nurturing food and habits into your life. Focus on what you want to eat because of how it makes you feel. Let the healthy crowd out the rest.

ACTION ITEM
Start to observe your food choices throughout the day with a curiosity mindset rather than an attitude of judgment. Later we will focus on more specifics. For now, observe your behavior without judgment or trying to change. You can also record your thoughts about what foods serve you well and those that do not.

Monday: _____

_____

_____

_____

_____

Tuesday: _____

_____

_____

_____

_____

Wednesday:_____

_____

_____

_____

_____

Thursday: _____

_____

_____

_____

_____

HEALTHY HABIT
CHECKLIST
☐ Remember where
you started & why
☐ Remember your
goals
☐ Drink water
☐ Add in to crowd out

Friday: _____

_____

_____

_____

_____

Saturday:_____

_____

_____

_____

_____

Sunday:_____

_____

_____

_____

_____

Weekly Summary: _____

_____

_____

_____

_____

_____

_____

_____

WEEK FIVE

"We should all be eating fruits and vegetables as if our life depended on it – because they do."
~Michael Gregor

Vegetables are packed with vitamins and minerals that are essential to helping us feel our best. Which vitamins and minerals, and the density, varies from plant to plant. Put very simply, your body is made up of many, many different systems. Different vitamins and minerals are essential for these systems to operate. What's more, for optimal function you need the right combination of a variety of different nutrients. In other words, you may need mineral A to create reaction B to synthesize C. If you don't get A, then you will not be able to synthesize C, which may be important for optimal sleep.

This is why it is important not just to consume many vegetables, but also to choose a variety of types, colors, and preparation methods. They will help to keep you healthy in the short run and long run. They will also make you feel better and have more energy.

For this week, begin by monitoring your current vegetable consumption. Then, if your diet is not largely vegetable based, start adding more. Aim for just one extra serving per day. This is a time to explore new things in order to find what works for you. Increase quantity and volume slowly over time as you adjust to a new way of eating. It will also take time to learn how to prepare new vegetables.

If you think you do not like vegetables, start trying them in different ways. Want a sweet treat? Roast squash, carrots, onion, and brussels sprouts in some oil and salt. Want to increase salad consumption at home? Find a homemade salad dressing recipe or just mix together olive oil, vinegar, Dijon mustard, pepper, and salt. Want to hide vegetables in meals you already eat? Add spinach or kale to a smoothie in the morning and start throwing added greens into soups and casseroles.

WEEK FIVE

Monday: _____

_____

_____

_____

_____

LESSON RECAP
Add in more vegetables for better short- and long-term health.

Tuesday: _____

_____

_____

_____

_____

ACTION ITEM
Eat at least one extra serving of vegetables each day this week and continue adding at a comfortable pace until they make up the bulk of your diet (by volume). Experiment with both quantity and variety. Record your experience as you explore new tastes.

Wednesday:_____

_____

_____

_____

_____

Thursday: _____

_____

_____

_____

_____

19

Friday: _____

HEALTHY HABIT CHECKLIST
□ Remember where you started & why
□ Remember your goals
□ Drink water
□ Add in to crowd out
□ Eat vegetables

_____
_____
_____
_____

Saturday:_____

_____
_____
_____
_____

Sunday:_____

_____
_____
_____
_____

Weekly Summary: _____

_____
_____
_____
_____
_____
_____
_____

WEEK SIX

"Eat Fat, Get Thin."
~Dr. Mark Hyman

Fat does not make you fat...so long as you are choosing the right types of fat to add to your diet. Fat is essential for your body to function optimally, including for brain health, regulating inflammation, hormone synthesis, and even for a healthy metabolism. In other words, you need fat to burn fat. Because many of us have heard for so long that we should avoid fat, it can be difficult to embrace the addition of healthy fats to a healthy diet. Be patient with yourself, but start looking at each meal and ensure that you are adding in healthy fats – and learn which ones to leave far behind.

Fats to add: Extra virgin olive oil, nut oils such as walnut or pecan, avocados and avocado oil, coconut oil, flaxseeds and flaxseed oil, nuts and seeds, sesame oil, butter, ghee, full-fat dairy.

Fats to avoid: Canola oil, vegetable oil, corn oil, soybean oil, safflower oil, margarine, hydrogenated or partially hydrogenated oils.

As a general rule, because the unhealthy fats are far cheaper, nearly every processed food item in the store is made with the unhealthy fats. Start reading labels and use this as a good reason to make the switch to whole foods – at a pace you are comfortable with.

For cooking: pay attention to the smoke point for oil. Stir frying with olive oil, for example, will probably exceed its smoke point, which makes it harmful. Avocado and coconut oils are both good for high-heat cooking; olive oil is excellent for salad dressings.

Monday: _____

_____

_____

_____

_____

LESSON RECAP
Fat is essential to a healthy diet and most of us are not eating enough. Focus on adding in high quality fats and replacing unhealthy fats.

Tuesday: _____

_____

_____

_____

_____

ACTION ITEM
Start by ensuring you are eating healthy fats every day, then begin incorporating them into each meal.

Wednesday:_____

_____

_____

_____

_____

Thursday: _____

_____

_____

_____

_____

Friday: _____

HEALTHY HABIT CHECKLIST
□ Remember where you started & why
□ Remember your goals
□ Drink water
□ Add in to crowd out
□ Eat vegetables
□ Eat healthy fats

_____

_____

_____

_____

Saturday:_____

_____

_____

_____

_____

Sunday:_____

_____

_____

_____

_____

Weekly Summary: _____

_____

_____

_____

_____

_____

_____

_____

30-DAY CHECK-IN POINT

REVISIT

In the following week, you will hit 30 days since Week Two, when you set goals for 30 days, 90 days, and 210 days. In addition to the weekly lesson and action item, take time in the next week to revisit the goals you established earlier. How are you doing on the goals you set? What have you accomplished? Do you want to change or eliminate any of the goals you wrote earlier? Are there goals you want to add? Timeframes you want to change?

Accomplishments so far using this journal: (Anything counts, even the things that seem *so small* are worth celebrating!)

_____

_____

_____

_____

Continued, modified, and new goals:
60 Days

1
_____

2
_____

3
_____

180 Days

1
_____

2
_____

3
_____

WEEK SEVEN

SLOWING IT DOWN

"If we are not fully ourselves, truly in the present moment, we miss everything."
~Thich Nhat Hanh

This week's focus is about bringing awareness to eating your food. This has two benefits. First, chewing is important for the start of the digestive process. Second, by paying attention to what you eat, you are more likely to eat less. How many times have you been snacking or eating while multi-tasking, only to realize with shock that you have eaten all that was in front of you, with little memory of the event?

Chewing starts the process of digestion. Not only does chewing play an essential role in breaking food down so that it can be processed through the stomach, intestines, and liver, but it also combines the food with the digestive enzymes in your mouth to begin the essential breakdown of food into the components that are useful to us. Some foods require that they be broken down by chewing in order to get the health benefits from them. For example, many greens contain anti-cancer compounds that can only be absorbed after chewing them. Aim to chew for 30 seconds per mouthful.

Slowing down is likely to lead to smaller meals because it allows your brain to register satiety before you have already overstuffed yourself. It's both a matter of actually being full and registering that fact, and feeling satisfied so that you do not keep munching.

This week, choose at least one meal per day and sit down to that meal. Do not eat standing up, in the car, or at your desk. Take a minute before eating to take a deep breath and transition to mealtime. Also consider your hunger level and how that feels in your stomach. Take a bite, put your fork or spoon down, and chew as many times as you can before there is nothing left to chew. Repeat throughout your meal. Pay attention to the different tastes and textures. After your meal, pay attention to how you feel differently than when you started.

WEEK SEVEN

Monday: _____
_____
_____
_____
_____

Tuesday: _____
_____
_____
_____

Wednesday:_____
_____
_____
_____

Thursday: _____
_____
_____
_____

LESSON RECAP
Chewing is essential to proper digestion and eating slowly helps to regulate how much and what you eat.

ACTION ITEM
Begin by focusing on one meal a day. Chew and devote your full attention to that meal (conversation is fine, but avoid TV and other screens). As the week and your life go on, continue paying attention to your meals by chewing and monitoring how they make you feel.

Friday: _____

**HEALTHY HABIT
CHECKLIST**
□ Remember where
you started & why
□ Remember your
goals
□ Drink water
□ Add in to crowd out
□ Eat vegetables
□ Eat healthy fats
□ Chew your food

Saturday:_____

Sunday:_____

Weekly Summary: _____

WEEK EIGHT

CRAVINGS AND HUNGER

"The less we indulge in something, the less we want it. When we believe that a craving will remain unsatisfied, it may diminish; cravings are more provoked by possibility than by denial."
~Gretchen Rubin

Cravings come on suddenly when we desire a particular food or type of food (sugar or salt for instance). It can feel like hunger, but often comes on quickly and you will feel like it can only be satisfied with particular things. Hunger, on the other hand, will develop slowly and you can feel it in your stomach. You will feel that a variety of foods will satisfy the hunger. Identifying the difference is important so that you know how to react to the feeling. The two can often be confused.

Cravings come in different forms. Sometimes it is our body telling us what we need more of in our diet. These are frequently milder cravings and lead you to desire a certain type of food, such as protein. This type of craving is important to listen to and can be satisfied with healthy food options.

Other cravings can be the opposite of our body's natural messaging. Sugar and fried foods fall into this category. These foods are addicting and when we eat them, we want more of them – this usually presents itself in the form of cravings. These cravings are best left alone or satisfied with a healthier option.

If you have cravings often, it may mean that you are lacking micronutrients in your diet. Focus on adding lots of plants with different colors into your diet. You may find that the cravings will go away naturally. It could also be emotional eating. Are you trying to hide something? What happens if you focus on the emotion instead of reaching for food? Cravings can also mean that you are dehydrated. You can see the interconnectedness between cravings and prior lessons. If you missed something or have forgotten prior lessons, this is a good time to go back and revisit. Stay simple and take small steps.

Monday: _____

_____

_____

_____

_____

Tuesday: _____

_____

_____

_____

_____

Wednesday:_____

_____

_____

_____

Thursday: _____

_____

_____

_____

LESSON RECAP
Cravings are different than hunger. This lesson teaches about the difference and what your cravings could be telling you.

ACTION ITEM
Start by monitoring. Are you truly hungry, or are you craving something that you do not need? What patterns do your cravings take? What happens when you avoid the food you crave for a few days? Do the cravings go away? Is the craving telling you something important about something missing from your diet?

Friday: _____

_____

_____

_____

_____

HEALTHY HABIT CHECKLIST
□ Remember where you started & why
□ Remember your goals
□ Drink water
□ Add in to crowd out
□ Eat vegetables
□ Eat healthy fats
□ Chew your food
□ Monitor cravings

Saturday:_____

_____

_____

_____

_____

Sunday:_____

_____

_____

_____

_____

Weekly Summary: _____

_____

_____

_____

_____

_____

_____

_____

WEEK NINE

"The gifts of imperfection: Let go of who you think you're supposed to be and embrace who you are."
~Brené Brown

Each of us is unique. We respond to foods differently, we each thrive on a different level of social interaction, our bodies do better with different forms of exercise, we enjoy different things, and we all find satisfaction at work in different ways. We also have different genes, different hormone levels, different allergies and tolerances, and different gut bacteria.

It would be easy to forget our inherent uniqueness because so many products treat individuals as though we are all the same. This is particularly true of the diet and fitness industry. Ads for the next great diet make it sound as if it will work for everyone. If a friend loses a bunch of weight using one strategy, and then we try it and don't lose weight, we may feel like a failure rather than recognizing that we are just a different person with a different make-up.

This concept is the most essential principle to finding the healthiest diet and lifestyle for you. That can be both empowering and frightening. Many of us want to be told exactly what to eat, yet because we are all unique, I cannot tell you what foods will be the best for you, and neither can anyone else. I can and will tell you to eat whole foods, with lots of vegetables and healthy fats. However, if you find that brussels sprouts do not make you feel good after eating them, then you should listen to your body and avoid them (no, this isn't an excuse not to eat them just because you do not like them).

Start to experiment to find out which way of eating works best for you. Use this program as a guide, and then trust your body to fine tune your happiest and healthiest life. Continually experiment, as you will change over time!

LESSON RECAP
Each of us has a unique way of eating that works best for our own body and mindset, as well as a unique best lifestyle. Trust your body to tell you what you need, and allow yourself to change at your own pace. You may find foods that don't make you feel great but which you love and are unwilling to go through life without. That's okay, and still important information to have.

ACTION ITEM
While using healthy eating principles in this program and your own experience as a guide, begin to listen to your body and experiment to discover the way of eating that works best for you.

Monday: _____

_____

_____

_____

_____

Tuesday: _____

_____

_____

_____

_____

Wednesday:_____

_____

_____

_____

_____

Thursday: _____

_____

_____

_____

_____

**HEALTHY HABIT
CHECKLIST**
☐ Remember where
you started & why
☐ Remember your
goals
☐ Drink water
☐ Add in to crowd out
☐ Eat vegetables
☐ Eat healthy fats
☐ Chew your food
☐ Monitor cravings
☐ Bioindividuality

Friday: _____

_____

_____

_____

_____

Saturday:_____

_____

_____

_____

_____

Sunday:_____

_____

_____

_____

_____

Weekly Summary: _____

_____

_____

_____

_____

_____

_____

_____

WEEK TEN

CAREER

"Burnout is not the price you have to pay for success."
~Arianna Huffington

Hopefully you love the work that you do. However, it may also be demanding, and it may have taken over your life. It is easy to get into a work routine and think that this is the way things must be. If you step back, you may find that small changes can make your work far more satisfying.

This week, take time to reflect on the work you do. Consider changes to make it fit you better.

Write out answers to these questions on a separate piece of paper, or work on it throughout the week in the space provided:

1. Do you define yourself by your career? Do you like your answer to this question?
2. What do you like and dislike most about your daily work?
3. If there were no barrier, no fear, no concern about money, what is one thing that you would change about how you spend your work hours?
4. Consider your answers to 1-3. What is one thing that you will do in the next week to improve your work environment? (This may be bringing a plant to work, rearranging your office, or deciding on a new approach to a troubling work relationship. Be creative: it's where you spend most of your time).
5. Then think bigger and long-term. What is one change that you want to have achieved in the next year to improve your work environment?

One helpful tool is to recognize your strengths in the workplace and to incorporate more work using those strengths. This is a good resource to help you do this: https://www.gallupstrengthscenter.com/

Monday: _____

_____

_____

_____

_____

LESSON RECAP
Work is likely where you spend most of your time. It is easy to become complacent. However, small changes in your environment and your behaviors could make a huge difference. What could your work-life look like?

Tuesday: _____

_____

_____

_____

_____

Wednesday:_____

_____

ACTION ITEM
Write out the answers to the five questions in this lesson and commit to short-term and long-term changes to improve your work environment. This isn't necessarily about career change; we all have room for improvement even if we love our current work.

_____

_____

_____

Thursday: _____

_____

_____

_____

_____

WEEK TEN

HEALTHY HABIT CHECKLIST

- ☐ Remember where you started & why
- ☐ Remember your goals
- ☐ Drink water
- ☐ Add in to crowd out
- ☐ Eat vegetables
- ☐ Eat healthy fats
- ☐ Chew your food
- ☐ Monitor cravings
- ☐ Bioindividuality
- ☐ Consider career

Friday: _____

_____

_____

_____

_____

Saturday: _____

_____

_____

_____

_____

Sunday: _____

_____

_____

_____

_____

Weekly Summary: _____

_____

_____

_____

_____

_____

_____

_____

WEEK ELEVEN

"We cannot become what we want by remaining what we are."
~Max de Pree

Routine is very, very powerful. When we do something every day, we no longer need to think about it. This can be true for anything, such as getting up at 5am to exercise, having a drink every day after work, cooking meals or eating out, or staying at your desk at lunch even though you keep promising yourself you will go to the gym.

When you want to make a change to your routine, it can help tremendously to be very conscious about how you go about developing this new habit. Here are a few tactics that have proven effective for some people. Know yourself and recognize that what works great for one person could activate your rebellious side and have the opposite effect on you. Try things out, and be patient with yourself if one way completely fails for you. If you want to change, and when you are ready, the new habit will stick.

1. Couple the new habit with a current habit. Want to drink a glass of water each morning? Do it before you brush your teeth.

2. Put it on your calendar. Want to exercise every day? Mark the precise time and what you will do on your calendar.

3. Set up an accountability system. Gyms, classes, personal trainers, health coaches, and friends might help keep you accountable. Simply announcing your goal may be enough, or paying for the gym membership, training session, or class. You could make a bet with a group of friends, or set up another reward system or a punishment if you do not do something.

4. Substitute. For example, drink Kombucha instead of your nightly alcoholic beverage.

LESSON RECAP
Developing new habits is challenging for anyone. There are many tricks that can help you create new, healthy habits. Here are a few ideas; keep trying different techniques until you find what will work for you.

ACTION ITEM
Think about one activity that you want to start doing and decide on one way that you are going to try to turn that activity into a habit. Get going. Stick with it, but if it doesn't work, try a new mechanism to change that activity into a habit.

Monday: _____

_____

_____

_____

_____

Tuesday: _____

_____

_____

_____

_____

Wednesday:_____

_____

_____

_____

_____

Thursday: _____

_____

_____

_____

_____

Friday: _____

_____

_____

_____

_____

HEALTHY HABIT CHECKLIST
□ Remember where you started & why
□ Remember your goals
□ Drink water
□ Add in to crowd out
□ Eat vegetables
□ Eat healthy fats
□ Chew your food
□ Monitor cravings
□ Bioindividuality
□ Consider career
□ New habits

Saturday:_____

_____

_____

_____

_____

Sunday:_____

_____

_____

_____

_____

Weekly Summary: _____

_____

_____

_____

_____

_____

_____

_____

WEEK TWELVE

PROBIOTICS

"A healthy outside starts from the inside."
~Robert Urich

We all have bacteria in our gut that help with the digestive process. Keeping these bacteria plentiful, happy, and healthy is very important to feeling our best. Eating fermented foods containing probiotics is a good way to increase the diversity and abundance of good bacteria in your gut.

Explore new tastes this week by choosing one of the following to eat each day and by exploring the biggest variety you can.

- Yogurt: I recommend whole-fat, plain yogurt because that fat is healthier than what they add in if the fat is removed, and plain because flavored options are usually packed with sugar. You can add your own fruit and even a little honey for some sweetness and flavor if you want.
- Kefir: A fermented milk drink found in most stores.
- Sauerkraut and pickles: Look for the varieties that are sold in the refrigerator section – make sure it says there are live probiotic cultures as many on the market do not have live probiotics.
- Kimchi
- Kombucha

Probiotics are undergoing a surge in popularity and you are likely to find a variety of different fermented foods and flavors at your local market. Experiment and find what you like. Add just a spoonful of the above to a meal for added flavor. You can also start making your own if you are so inclined. Find directions for fermented foods online or elsewhere; you can also purchase kits with the tools to get you started.

Monday: _____

_____

_____

LESSON RECAP
Probiotic foods are
a healthy, daily
addition to your
diet. They will
increase the
prevalence of
healthy gut
bacteria which
help with digestion
and overall health.

Tuesday: _____

_____

_____

_____

ACTION ITEM
Explore as many
new probiotic
foods this week as
you can. Take a
trip to the grocery
store and try both
exciting and scary
things. You may
develop surprising
tastes.

Wednesday:_____

_____

_____

_____

Thursday: _____

_____

_____

_____

HEALTHY HABIT CHECKLIST
- ☐ Remember where you started & why
- ☐ Remember your goals
- ☐ Drink water
- ☐ Add in to crowd out
- ☐ Eat vegetables
- ☐ Eat healthy fats
- ☐ Chew your food
- ☐ Monitor cravings
- ☐ Bioindividuality
- ☐ Consider career
- ☐ New habits
- ☐ Probiotics

Friday: _____

_____

_____

_____

_____

Saturday: _____

_____

_____

_____

_____

Sunday: _____

_____

_____

_____

_____

Weekly Summary: _____

_____

_____

_____

_____

_____

_____

_____

WEEK THIRTEEN

QUIET CONNECTION

"All courses of action are risky, so prudence is not in avoiding danger (it's impossible), but calculating risk and acting decisively. Make mistakes of ambition and not mistakes of sloth. Develop the strength to do bold things, not the strength to suffer."
~Niccolo Machiavelli

Developing practices to connect to something outside of ourselves can help us live our best lives. This resonates differently for different people. For some, it is a deep spiritual or religious practice. It could also be meditation, a regular habit to get out into nature, or reading inspirational pieces or poetry. Quiet connection with something outside of yourself may also mean regularly volunteering your time to help others or a cause you care about.

If this isn't already a part of your life, give some thought to what speaks to you and plan to incorporate it into your life. You may need to try different things. For example, there are many types of meditation that work better for different people. To get started you could simply focus on your breath for a minute each day. Or consider getting started with an app such as Headspace or Calm, or going more in depth with a meditation course. Ziva Meditation or Transcendental Meditation are popular options differing in their approach.

If you already have a practice of quiet connection, what are one or two things you can put into place this week to strengthen your practice?

These are all easy pieces to let slide in our busy lives, but slowing down and meaningfully connecting with something outside of yourself and your immediate world will actually benefit those around you and yourself by allowing you to be more present with the world you live in.

Monday: _____

LESSON RECAP
An important part
of taking care of
yourself is to
spend time in
reflection and
considering the
world outside of
your immediate
environment.

_____
_____
_____
_____

Tuesday: _____

_____
_____
_____

ACTION ITEM
Reflect on your
current practices
of quiet
connection. If you
already have a
practice, what can
you start this week
to strengthen your
connection? If you
do not have a
practice, what
interests you? Do
you want to try
meditation? Spend
more quiet time in
nature? Use this
week to explore. It
may take time to
find the practice
that resonates
with you the most.

Wednesday:_____

_____
_____
_____
_____

Thursday: _____

_____
_____
_____
_____

Friday: _____

HEALTHY HABIT
CHECKLIST
□ Remember where
you started & why
□ Remember your
goals
□ Drink water
□ Add in to crowd out
□ Eat vegetables
□ Eat healthy fats
□ Chew your food
□ Monitor cravings
□ Bioindividuality
□ Consider career
□ New habits
□ Probiotics
□ Quiet connection

Saturday:_____

Sunday:_____

Weekly Summary: _____

WEEK FOURTEEN

INCORPORATE DAILY MOVEMENT

"Exercise is honest, inexpensive, all-natural medicine. It's also the easiest, cheapest, and fastest way to a happy life."
~Jordan D. Metzl, M.D.

Exercise has long-term benefits: it can help prevent chronic disease, reduces your risk of developing Alzheimer's, may increase longevity and decrease your risk of developing cancer, reduces inflammation, helps to regulate blood sugar levels, is helpful to brain health, and it has been shown to be as effective as medication for some people in treating depression. Exercise also has more immediate benefits you may feel right away: it boosts mood, increases concentration, increases dopamine – a motivation hormone – improves sleep, reduces anxiety, and increases self-discipline.

If you do not currently exercise regularly, start focusing on moving more every day. It doesn't have to be fancy. Add activity slowly. If you cannot find something you really like to do, commit to movement that you will do in such small increments that you will stick with it.

If you already exercise, look at what you are doing. Do you want to make an improvement, such as adding a strength program to what you are already doing? Or incorporate something to liven it?

Studies show that increasing effort in short bursts is more beneficial to overall fitness than steady state. Thus, if you find 15 minutes per day for a walk, after a few minutes of movement, increase the pace for 2 minutes, and then ease back for 1 minute, and repeat this pattern until your walk is over. If you can devote more than 15 minutes per day, find something you love to do. Dance, yoga, swimming – experiment and find something you enjoy, then make it a habit! Starting new exercise in a group is one of the biggest fears people have. Remember that everyone has this fear. Ask for help, and after the first time or two, the fear will probably go away.

LESSON RECAP
Movement is good for both long- and short-term health. Even if you are not able to be 'perfect' and get to the gym every day, you can do tremendous good by just moving your body.

ACTION ITEM
Take a realistic assessment of your current movement. Not just exercise, but how often you move throughout the day. Decide on one or two things to incorporate immediately to increase your level of movement and implement this week.

Monday: _____

_____

_____

_____

_____

Tuesday: _____

_____

_____

_____

_____

Wednesday:_____

_____

_____

_____

_____

Thursday: _____

_____

_____

_____

_____

Friday: _____

_____

_____

_____

_____

HEALTHY HABIT CHECKLIST
- ☐ Remember where you started & why
- ☐ Remember your goals
- ☐ Drink water
- ☐ Add in to crowd out
- ☐ Eat vegetables
- ☐ Eat healthy fats
- ☐ Chew your food
- ☐ Monitor cravings
- ☐ Bioindividuality
- ☐ Consider career
- ☐ New habits
- ☐ Probiotics
- ☐ Quiet connection
- ☐ Move your body

Saturday:_____

_____

_____

_____

_____

Sunday:_____

_____

_____

_____

_____

Weekly Summary: _____

_____

_____

_____

_____

_____

_____

_____

WEEK FIFTEEN

"You must do the thing you think you cannot do."
~Eleanor Roosevelt

This may be the week you have been dreading, but it is one of the most important. Added sugar is one of the worst things we can consume. It alters our internal chemistry, leaving us in a haze with our internal sense of what is healthy skewed. Overconsumption of sugar can lead to fatigue, depression, mood swings, weight gain, insulin resistance, type 2 diabetes, heart disease, and cancer.

What is too much and what can you do about it? There are naturally occurring sugars in foods such as fruit and dairy products. These are not addressed here. Rather, consider added sugars which can be found in a lot of processed foods, sweet treats, and added directly to food and drinks. The American Heart Association recommends the following daily limits of added sugars: no more than 25 grams of added sugar per day for women, and 36 grams for men. Some labels will indicate what amount of sugar is added. If a label does not indicate added sugar, generally assume that any sugar in a processed food item will be added (with the exception of plain whole milk and yogurt).

While some sweeteners such as honey, maple syrup, and molasses are better options than refined white sugar because of their higher nutrient content, they still count as added sugars to your diet.

Do not make the mistake of switching to artificial sweeteners such as saccharin or aspartame – often found in diet sodas. These sweeteners can lead to weight gain and are stored by our bodies as toxins.

Determine which foods in your home contain the most sugar. Pay attention to ketchup, yogurt, cereal, spaghetti sauce, bread, processed meat, BBQ sauce, juices, crackers, and of course the sweet items where you would expect to find it. For many options you can find better alternatives, such as spaghetti sauce without added sugar.

LESSON RECAP
Added sugar is one of the worst things we can put in our bodies, yet it is everywhere. Start paying attention to labels, and make sure not to replace with artificial sweeteners.

ACTION ITEM
Look at the items in your home to find the added sugars. Start paying attention to labels when at the grocery store. For the next few days, start calculating your total grams of added sugar per day so that you know where you stand, and then begin to reduce if needed. Sugar is addicting and change may take time. Be patient with yourself but know that reducing sugar is one of the best things you can do for your health.

Monday: _____

_____

_____

_____

_____

Tuesday: _____

_____

_____

_____

_____

Wednesday:_____

_____

_____

_____

_____

Thursday: _____

_____

_____

_____

_____

HEALTHY HABIT
CHECKLIST
☐ Remember where
you started & why
☐ Remember your
goals
☐ Drink water
☐ Add in to crowd out
☐ Eat vegetables
☐ Eat healthy fats
☐ Chew your food
☐ Monitor cravings
☐ Bioindividuality
☐ Consider career
☐ New habits
☐ Probiotics
☐ Quiet connection
☐ Move your body
☐ Sugar

Friday: _____

_____

_____

_____

_____

Saturday:_____

_____

_____

_____

Sunday:_____

_____

_____

_____

_____

Weekly Summary: _____

_____

_____

_____

_____

_____

_____

_____

HALFWAY POINT

In the following week you will hit 90 days since Week Two when you set goals for 30 days, 90 days, and 210 days. It is also your halfway point. In addition to the weekly lesson and action item, take time in the next week to revisit the goals you established earlier. How are you doing on the goals you set? What have you accomplished? Do you want to change or eliminate any of the goals you established earlier? Are there goals you want to add? Timeframes you want to change?

Also revisit the Circle of Life on the following page. Do it before reviewing the one you completed in week one, but then go back to compare.

Accomplishments so far using this journal: (Anything counts, even the things that seem *so small* are worth celebrating!)

_____

_____

_____

_____

_____

_____

Continued, modified, and new goals:
120 Days

1
_____

2
_____

3
_____

CIRCLE OF LIFE

Complete the circle of life again at this point in your journey: Place a dot in the wedge for each category to indicate your level of satisfaction in that area. The center of the circle indicates zero satisfaction in that area; the outer edge indicates complete satisfaction in that area. Satisfaction means you do not feel there is room for improvement at this time in your life. Focus only on how you feel at this time. For example, education may not play a big role in your life right now, but if you are completely satisfied and do not wish to increase its role at this time, then you would put your dot near the outer edge of the circle. When you are done, connect the dots.

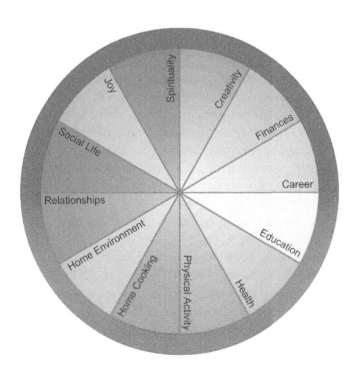

WEEK SIXTEEN

"Do your own thinking independently. Be the chess player, not the chess piece."
~Ralph Charell

For many healthy people, grains are a staple of their diet. Meanwhile, many others feel better without any grains at all. What's best for you is something you need to decide for yourself. However, there is no question that if you eat grains, they should be whole and intact. This is because whole grains take much longer to digest than highly processed grains (including whole grains ground up into flours), which are quickly digested. This causes insulin to spike and then crash, which in turn will make you feel hungrier and crave less-healthy foods that will quickly get your insulin levels back up.

Products can be labeled "whole grain" even when they contain mostly refined grains that have the nutritious bran and germ removed. Therefore, it is best to consume grains that you have cooked yourself or that appear intact – brown rice or a store-bought quinoa salad, for example. Other good options to include in your diet are kasha, millet, and steel-cut oats (these are better than regular oats, but regular is fine if you prefer it; avoid quick-cooking oats).

Whole grains can take a long time to cook, and you are busy. Fortunately, they save well and can be reused for many meals. You could make a huge pot of brown rice one evening for a curry, and then use it for stir-fried rice later in the week and atop salads for lunches. Or make a large pot of steel-cut oats as a breakfast cereal over the weekend, and eat it throughout the week. Once you get into the habit, even the busiest person can find ways to incorporate healthy, whole grains. If you are not ready to give up bread (made of highly-processed flour), look for sprouted-grain breads that will contain the actual whole grains.

LESSON RECAP
Grains can be incorporated into a healthy diet (though some people feel better without them), but avoid processed grains in favor of whole, intact grains.

ACTION ITEM
Two options this week: 1) Bring awareness to your choices and begin adding in more truly whole grains. Try one grain this week that you have never cooked before. 2) Alternatively, go grain-free this week. Focus on healthy fats, protein, and vegetables instead. Go at least one week, perhaps two, before you decide whether grain-free living makes you feel better. If it feels right, stick with it, if you feel better with grains, now you know.

Monday: _____

_____

_____

_____

_____

Tuesday: _____

_____

_____

_____

_____

Wednesday:_____

_____

_____

_____

_____

Thursday: _____

_____

_____

_____

_____

Friday: _____

_____

_____

_____

_____

HEALTHY HABIT
CHECKLIST
☐ Remember where
you started & why
☐ Remember your
goals
☐ Drink water
☐ Add in to crowd out
☐ Eat vegetables
☐ Eat healthy fats
☐ Chew your food
☐ Monitor cravings
☐ Bioindividuality
☐ Consider career
☐ New habits
☐ Probiotics
☐ Quiet connection
☐ Move your body
☐ Sugar
☐ Whole grains

Saturday:_____

_____

_____

_____

_____

Sunday:_____

_____

_____

_____

_____

Weekly Summary: _____

_____

_____

_____

_____

_____

_____

_____

WEEK SEVENTEEN

SLEEP

"Fatigue makes cowards of us all."
~George S. Patton Jr.

Sleep fuels so much of our body's functioning. It's during sleep that our bodies repair themselves, detox from unwanted substances during the day, and generally reset. Without solid sleep, our bodies can't function to their full potential no matter how we eat and exercise. Furthermore, if you have sufficient sleep, you are much more likely to fit in exercise and to eat well. We all need somewhere between 7-9 hours of sleep per night, and you cannot sleep less during the week and make up for it on the weekends. If you continually get less and think that you are one of the lucky ones who can function on 5 hours a night, in all likelihood, you are not. You are probably just used to functioning sub-optimally. You may be lucky: perhaps your optimal function is a really high bar, so you are doing great at sub-par. But you will feel better, get more done, and improve your life if you start to prioritize sleep. You may attempt to sleep 7-9 hours per night and have trouble falling asleep or staying asleep. You are not alone. This is very common, but not a reason not to try new techniques to break through the barrier.

Here are some tips to help you get 7-9 hours of solid sleep per night:
- Set a bedtime and try to keep it consistent throughout the week (including weekends).
- Develop a bedtime routine. This may include a cup of tea, putting on your favorite pajamas, or reading a book. Try to avoid looking at screens for at least 60 minutes before your bedtime (two hours is ideal), and consider blue-light blocking glasses before then.
- Take care in setting up your sleeping space. It should be dark and free of distractions, with bedding you love.
- Avoid caffeine in the afternoon.
- Stop eating at least two hours (the more the better) before your bedtime.
- Exercise during the day and eat a healthy diet.

Monday: _____

_____

_____

_____

_____

LESSON RECAP
Sleep is the foundation to a healthy, vibrant life. Without good sleep, other habits are difficult to maintain and they will not make as much of a difference.

Tuesday: _____

_____

_____

_____

_____

ACTION ITEM
If you do not get between 7-9 hours of sleep per night, figure out how you can do it. Take a look at your day's schedule and find a way to adjust it. Then, whether you get 7-9 hours per night or not, try one or two practices this week to see if they will improve your sleep quality.

Wednesday:_____

_____

_____

_____

_____

Thursday: _____

_____

_____

_____

_____

HEALTHY HABIT CHECKLIST
- ☐ Remember where you started & why
- ☐ Remember your goals
- ☐ Drink water
- ☐ Add in to crowd out
- ☐ Eat vegetables
- ☐ Eat healthy fats
- ☐ Chew your food
- ☐ Monitor cravings
- ☐ Bioindividuality
- ☐ Consider career
- ☐ New habits
- ☐ Probiotics
- ☐ Quiet connection
- ☐ Move your body
- ☐ Sugar
- ☐ Whole grains
- ☐ Sleep

Friday: _____

_____

_____

_____

_____

Saturday:_____

_____

_____

_____

_____

Sunday:_____

_____

_____

_____

_____

Weekly Summary: _____

_____

_____

_____

_____

_____

_____

_____

WEEK EIGHTEEN

"If you keep good food in your fridge, you'll eat good food."
~Errick McAdams

While we are all bioindividuals who will do best eating a slightly different diet, the one constant is that we should all strive to eat mostly whole, real food. Currently, the American diet is largely made up of processed foods, many of which our bodies do not even recognize as food at all. Because we think of these items as food, it can take time to transition to a diet based on real ingredients. It may require a shift in the way you approach grocery shopping, planning meals, and choosing what to eat at a restaurant.

What does it mean to avoid processed foods? Here are a few guidelines to get you started:

1. Consider the number of ingredients. If there is only one ingredient, it is probably a whole food item, such as grapes, carrots, tofu, chicken breast, or rice.

2. Can you recognize all the ingredients? Look for items that you can pronounce and recognize. Peanut butter may come with added salt, but avoid it if it has other additives such as added oil or other unrecognizable ingredients.

3. Does it belong? Items like ketchup and spaghetti sauce often contain added sugar. There is no need for sugar in such savory items, so try to avoid products with sugar if it shouldn't be there, or if they contain other odd ingredients that are not necessary.

There are some common items that are processed and which do not have great alternatives. Try to reduce or avoid these items, such as crackers, bread, and chips. Think up new snacks and easy meals instead. Don't overhaul all at once: small modifications will lead to a diet overhaul with time.

LESSON RECAP

We should all try to avoid processed foods. Instead, learn to shop for and cook with real food - single ingredient items that can be combined into delicious meals or enjoyed on their own.

ACTION ITEM

Begin by becoming aware of what you are consuming and purchasing. Start choosing store items with fewer or cleaner ingredients that you can pronounce. Then consider not replacing some processed staples in your home. For example, don't restock the chips, and try out new snacks such as nuts or vegetables and hummus for your family.

Monday: _____

_____

_____

_____

_____

Tuesday: _____

_____

_____

_____

_____

Wednesday:_____

_____

_____

_____

Thursday: _____

_____

_____

_____

HEALTHY HABIT CHECKLIST
- ☐ Remember where you started & why
- ☐ Remember your goals
- ☐ Drink water
- ☐ Add in to crowd out
- ☐ Eat vegetables
- ☐ Eat healthy fats
- ☐ Chew your food
- ☐ Monitor cravings
- ☐ Bioindividuality
- ☐ Consider career
- ☐ New habits
- ☐ Probiotics
- ☐ Quiet connection
- ☐ Move your body
- ☐ Sugar
- ☐ Whole grains
- ☐ Sleep
- ☐ No processed food

Friday: _____

_____

_____

_____

_____

Saturday:_____

_____

_____

_____

_____

Sunday:_____

_____

_____

_____

_____

Weekly Summary: _____

_____

_____

_____

_____

_____

_____

_____

WEEK NINETEEN

*"The man who has anticipated the coming of troubles takes away their
power when they arrive."*
~Seneca

Eating home-cooked meals does not have to be time consuming. Nor
does food preparation for the week have to entail a half day or more in
the kitchen. It doesn't have to be perfect, and it may take time to learn,
but investing a little time can have an important impact on your overall
health. Here are some techniques to make eating at home easier:

1. Plan to have the same basic ingredients around to use each week so
that shopping becomes easier and you have a basic idea of what you
will prepare that week. You can tweak your list if you want to get
certain ingredients for a particular recipe, but this way you will have
fewer decisions to make each week. To start, plan out three meals and
buy a little extra of the ingredients to use in other dishes that you think
up as you go.

2. Cook once, and eat twice (or more). When making any meal, make
more than a single meal's worth so that you have leftovers. If you get
tired of foods quickly, freeze some for later and cycle through. You can
also prepare more of a certain ingredient to use for later – make a huge
batch of rice and use it for different meals and different dishes, such as
fried rice or a rice pudding for dessert or breakfast.

3. A good way to have healthy snacks and desserts on hand is to make a
big batch of homemade items and freeze them. Consider some healthy
muffins, zucchini or pumpkin bread, or some low-sugar cookies that you
can make ahead of time and freeze.

4. To make simple meals that will satisfy the whole family, spend time
creating a Lazy Susan full of spices to keep on your kitchen table. This
way everyone in the family can choose how they want to season their
own meal.

Monday: _____

_____

_____

_____

_____

Tuesday: _____

_____

_____

_____

_____

Wednesday:_____

_____

_____

_____

_____

Thursday: _____

_____

_____

_____

_____

LESSON RECAP
Eating home-cooked meals is generally healthier than store-bought or restaurant meals and it doesn't have to run your life if you learn simple techniques to make cooking easy and satisfying.

ACTION ITEM
Choose one of these techniques to try out this week. Then reflect on how it went and set another short-term goal for yourself. Think of small things you can tweak to make eating home-cooked meals just a little easier. Don't do it all at once, but remain diligent and with time you can create more efficiency and enjoyment around home-cooked meals.

Friday: _____

_____

_____

_____

_____

HEALTHY HABIT CHECKLIST
- Remember where you started & why
- Remember your goals
- Drink water
- Add in to crowd out
- Eat vegetables
- Eat healthy fats
- Chew your food
- Monitor cravings
- Bioindividuality
- Consider career
- New habits
- Probiotics
- Quiet connection
- Move your body
- Sugar
- Whole grains
- Sleep
- No processed food
- Home-cooked meals

Saturday: _____

_____

_____

_____

_____

Sunday: _____

_____

_____

_____

_____

Weekly Summary: _____

_____

_____

_____

_____

_____

_____

_____

WEEK TWENTY

"Let gratitude be the pillow upon which you kneel to say your nightly prayer."
~Maya Angelou

While it may seem counterintuitive, a large part of being happy comes from how we think about our own lives and the world around us. Simply focusing on what is going well can alter how you see your world and how happy you are on a daily basis. If every day you write down something that you are grateful for, you will eventually start to look for the positive throughout your day, rather than highlighting the negative as we are prone to do.

Every one of us has blessings in our lives, but we often don't acknowledge them, so we become fixated on what we don't have and we end up missing what we do have. We become stressed for almost no reason because we can't see the bounty we have already earned!

This week, at the end of each day, write out three things for which you are grateful. These can be small things or big things. Just write them down and acknowledge them. Do this regularly for a week. You are likely to find that your thoughts will start to become happier and more positive.

After this week, consider if this is something you want to keep up, and if not, how might you change it. Should you write in the morning instead? Incorporate gratitude into a meditation practice? Write out three things just before leaving work for the day? Make it your own, and continue to see what happens.

Monday: _____

_____

_____

_____

_____

LESSON RECAP
By focusing on what we have rather than what we do not have, we can change how we see the world and our overall happiness.

Tuesday: _____

_____

_____

_____

_____

ACTION ITEM
Each evening, write out three things that you are grateful for. Don't overthink it; they can be small or big. However, be specific in your thoughts. If you are grateful for a person or a pet, what's one thing about them you are grateful for? It is okay to repeat items throughout the week, but still be sure to write three each day.

Wednesday:_____

_____

_____

_____

_____

Thursday: _____

_____

_____

_____

_____

HEALTHY HABIT CHECKLIST
- Remember where you started & why
- Remember your goals
- Drink water
- Add in to crowd out
- Eat vegetables
- Eat healthy fats
- Chew your food
- Monitor cravings
- Bioindividuality
- Consider career
- New habits
- Probiotics
- Quiet connection
- Move your body
- Sugar
- Whole grains
- Sleep
- No processed food
- Home-cooked meals
- Gratitude

Friday: _____

_____

_____

_____

_____

Saturday:_____

_____

_____

_____

Sunday:_____

_____

_____

_____

Weekly Summary: _____

_____

_____

_____

_____

_____

_____

WEEK TWENTY-ONE

EATING OUT

"When you know what's important, it's a lot easier to ignore what's not."
~Marie Forleo

It is harder to be as in control of what we consume when eating out, but dining at a restaurant is something that you probably do at least occasionally, and perhaps very regularly for work or out of habit. When eating out, there are many ways that you can get a healthier meal. Consider these:

1. Restaurant portions are often very large. Decide when you get your meal to eat half and save the rest for later. Make the division immediately so that you do not find yourself eating the whole meal without thinking.

2. Order one or two healthy appetizers instead of an entree.

3. Decide what you want to eat before entering the restaurant. Do not even look at the menu. Do you want a salad? Or chicken with rice and broccoli? Tell your server what you want to eat and they can direct you to different options. Often the chef will be happy to create the meal that you want even if it isn't on the menu (and particularly if it is simple).

4. Ask for your food to be cooked using olive oil instead of vegetable oil.

5. Ask for more vegetables instead of a starch, or consider a lettuce bun instead of bread, or a burrito without the tortilla, etc.

6. Be careful with the alcohol, particularly mixed drinks that are full of sugar. Consider nursing one or two drinks all evening.

7. And sometimes, make dining out a special occasion: order something special and enjoy the heck out of your meal.

69

WEEK TWENTY-ONE

Monday: _____

_____

_____

_____

_____

LESSON RECAP
Eating out can mean losing control of the quality of ingredients used and can lead you to eat portions far greater than necessary. However, with some planning and conscious decision making, it can be made a healthier, if still not a good regular choice.

Tuesday: _____

_____

_____

_____

_____

Wednesday:_____

_____

_____

_____

_____

ACTION ITEM
Try at least one of these tips the next time you eat a meal out.

Thursday: _____

_____

_____

_____

_____

HEALTHY HABIT CHECKLIST

☐ Remember where you started & why
☐ Remember your goals
☐ Drink water
☐ Add in to crowd out
☐ Eat vegetables
☐ Eat healthy fats
☐ Chew your food
☐ Monitor cravings
☐ Bioindividuality
☐ Consider career
☐ New habits
☐ Probiotics
☐ Quiet connection
☐ Move your body
☐ Sugar
☐ Whole grains
☐ Sleep
☐ No processed food
☐ Home-cooked meals
☐ Gratitude
☐ Eating out

Friday: _____

_____

_____

_____

_____

Saturday:_____

_____

_____

_____

Sunday:_____

_____

_____

_____

Weekly Summary: _____

_____

_____

_____

_____

_____

_____

_____

WEEK TWENTY-TWO

CHOOSING YOUR RELATIONSHIPS WISELY

"You're the average of the five people you spend the most time with."
~Jim Rohn

You are influenced by the people around you. This is true for all of us in both negative and positive ways. Studies show that you are more likely to eat better if those around you do, and the same goes for exercise habits. Yet it runs much deeper than just our behaviors. We are social creatures, and our relationships are deeply important to who we are as individuals. Even the most introverted among us do not live in a vacuum away from human interactions.

Consider who you spend your time with. Do you have at least one close friend you can turn to when you are struggling with something? How do you feel when you do turn to them? Do they make you feel down on yourself, or do they ask you questions that help you reflect and work through the problem in a helpful manner? How are you as a friend? Do you make time to listen and help others when they are in need? Are you present with those around you, or are you thinking about what to say next when you talk to someone?

Relationships do not just happen. They take conscious effort. This isn't something we are taught in school. It is easy to look at others and think they have a natural ability, but even the most polished individual may also feel a little vulnerable when inviting a new friend over for a meal.

This week, consider your current relationships. Choose at least one to focus on this week. This could mean one relationship you want to strengthen, or one that you want to let go because it doesn't serve you. Write out the action steps you will take and then execute.

LESSON RECAP
Relationships are
important no
matter what you
do, who you are,
or how introverted
you may be. Take a
good, honest look
at your current
relationships.

ACTION ITEM
Spend time this
week reflecting on
your relationships.
Then decide on at
least one that you
want to foster or
one that you want
to let go. Come up
with at least one
concrete thing that
you will do in
furtherance of a
change in that
relationship (such
as a way to reach
out to an
individual to do
something or a
strategy for telling
someone that you
wish to spend less
time with them).

Monday: _____

_____

_____

_____

_____

Tuesday: _____

_____

_____

_____

_____

Wednesday:_____

_____

_____

_____

_____

Thursday: _____

_____

_____

_____

_____

HEALTHY HABIT CHECKLIST
☐ Remember where you started & why
☐ Remember your goals
☐ Drink water
☐ Add in to crowd out
☐ Eat vegetables
☐ Eat healthy fats
☐ Chew your food
☐ Monitor cravings
☐ Bioindividuality
☐ Consider career
☐ New habits
☐ Probiotics
☐ Quiet connection
☐ Move your body
☐ Sugar
☐ Whole grains
☐ Sleep
☐ No processed food
☐ Home-cooked meals
☐ Gratitude
☐ Eating out
☐ Relationships

Friday: _____

_____

_____

_____

_____

Saturday: _____

_____

_____

_____

_____

Sunday: _____

_____

_____

_____

_____

Weekly Summary: _____

_____

_____

_____

_____

_____

_____

_____

WEEK TWENTY-THREE

Vitamin D

"Sunshine almost always makes me high."
~John Denver

Vitamin D, which we primarily receive from the sun, is incredibly important to our health. It's key to developing strong bones, healthy skin, and maintaining a positive mindset. It helps strengthen our immune system, produce hormones, and balance our energy levels and mood. Our bodies need natural sunlight, and let's face it, what is better than feeling its warmth on a nice day?

We are all different in how well we absorb vitamin D from the sunshine and how much we are able to get in our daily lives. It's a great idea to get your vitamin D levels checked regularly, and to supplement it if needed.

In the meantime, try to get a little bit of natural sunlight each day, taking precautions by wearing sunscreen, appropriate clothing, a hat, and eye protection. Try to soak up natural light whenever and however you can! It's important to take advantage of the natural wellness opportunities nature offers us.

If you live in a place with very little sun, try using a sunlamp to reap the benefits indoors as well as getting outdoors even if the sun isn't actively shining.

Monday: _____

_____

_____

_____

_____

LESSON RECAP
Vitamin D is important for optimal health. Try to get natural sunlight each day.

Tuesday: _____

_____

_____

_____

ACTION ITEM
If you do not get much sunlight, start making an effort to be in the sunshine every day it's out. Step outside your office for a small sunshine break; it will boost your mood and productivity later in the day. If this isn't an option in your region of the world, get a special lamp and use as directed.

Wednesday:_____

_____

_____

_____

Thursday: _____

_____

_____

_____

_____

HEALTHY HABIT CHECKLIST

☐ Remember where you started & why
☐ Remember your goals
☐ Drink water
☐ Add in to crowd out
☐ Eat vegetables
☐ Eat healthy fats
☐ Chew your food
☐ Monitor cravings
☐ Bioindividuality
☐ Consider career
☐ New habits
☐ Probiotics
☐ Quiet connection
☐ Move your body
☐ Sugar
☐ Whole grains
☐ Sleep
☐ No processed food
☐ Home-cooked meals
☐ Gratitude
☐ Eating out
☐ Relationships
☐ Vitamin D

Friday: _____

_____

_____

_____

_____

Saturday:_____

_____

_____

_____

_____

Sunday:_____

_____

_____

_____

_____

Weekly Summary: _____

_____

_____

_____

_____

_____

_____

_____

WEEK TWENTY-FOUR

MEAT

"You are what you eat. But also what your food eats."
~Ariel Goldenberg

Whether you choose to eat meat is a personal choice based on how you feel consuming different types of meat, as well as ethical or environmental concerns. If you choose not to eat meat based on ethical or environmental reasons, and yet find yourself feeling weak or out of sorts, consider experimenting with a small amount of meat or fish to see if it changes how you feel. Similarly, if you have always eaten meat, consider cutting it out this week to see how you feel without it. Many people report feeling better and losing weight easily on a plant-based diet but many people experience the same results on a meat-based diet. It depends on your own body, and you will not know until you try, or re-try if you experimented with different levels of meat long ago.

If you do choose to eat meat, your choices can have a huge impact on your health. The diet and health conditions of the animals you eat have an effect on the nutritional value of that meat.

Choose grass-fed beef. This will be labeled as such. It may be harder to find and will be more expensive, but it is worth it. This beef will have a much better fat profile (more omega-3 fats) than grain-fed beef, and will contain far more essential nutrients. Choose chicken that is organic. In the U.S. this will also mean that the chicken has not been fed antibiotics or arsenic. Free-range or pasture-raised are good options too.

Labeling in the U.S. can be vague. If you can, choose local meat from someone you can talk to and learn about how the animals were treated and what they were fed. You might find good, healthy meat options that are not labeled as above. Getting the appropriate government label can be an expensive process for the producer, but if you can meet the local farmer and find out how the animal was raised, that can be sufficient.

Monday: _____

LESSON RECAP
Whether or not you choose to eat meat is a personal decision. However, if you do elect to eat meat, choosing grass-fed beef or organic chicken is healthier than conventional meat.

_____

_____

_____

_____

Tuesday: _____

_____

_____

_____

_____

ACTION ITEM
If you do eat meat, or want to try adding it back in, then pick something to explore this week. That might mean not eating it, trying a new type, or trying grass-fed beef. If you do not eat meat, pick another goal for the week, perhaps continuing something from a prior lesson.

Wednesday:_____

_____

_____

_____

_____

Thursday: _____

_____

_____

_____

_____

HEALTHY HABIT CHECKLIST

☐ Remember where you started & why
☐ Remember your goals
☐ Drink water
☐ Add in to crowd out
☐ Eat vegetables
☐ Eat healthy fats
☐ Chew your food
☐ Monitor cravings
☐ Bioindividuality
☐ Consider career
☐ New habits
☐ Probiotics
☐ Quiet connection
☐ Move your body
☐ Sugar
☐ Whole grains
☐ Sleep
☐ No processed food
☐ Home-cooked meals
☐ Gratitude
☐ Eating out
☐ Relationships
☐ Vitamin D
☐ Meat

Friday: _____

_____

_____

_____

_____

Saturday:_____

_____

_____

_____

_____

Sunday:_____

_____

_____

_____

_____

Weekly Summary: _____

_____

_____

_____

_____

_____

_____

_____

WEEK TWENTY-FIVE

DAIRY

*"We should not, like sheep, follow the herd of creatures in front of us,
making our way where others go, not where we ought to go."*
~Seneca

Over 60% of adults are lactose intolerant, meaning that they cannot digest the sugar found in milk products. Symptoms of intolerance can include bloating, gas, abdominal pain, nausea, indigestion, diarrhea, and chronic stuffy nose and mucus. People can be affected by some dairy products but not others, or can consume a small amount without any side effects. This can have to do with your body's ability to digest a certain amount, or the nature of the product itself: some yogurt and cheese, for example, is made in a way that largely breaks down the lactose through fermentation.

Even if you do not recognize the symptoms, you could be experiencing some negative effects of dairy consumption without realizing it. This week, try cutting out dairy (including milk, cheese, butter, and yogurt) completely from your diet to see how you feel. Then begin adding dairy back in, one type (i.e. cheese, yogurt, or milk) at a time to monitor symptoms. You will need to experiment to learn what makes you feel your best.

If you do consume dairy products, aim for organic, whole-fat, and plain.

If you find that you feel better without dairy, there are substitutes on the market, including almond, coconut, or rice milk, and soy or cashew yogurt. Coconut oil and ghee can usually serve as a good substitute for butter. There are dairy-free cheese alternatives. They don't taste quite the same but you can experiment with them, or leave cheese out altogether. You might also choose to continue eating dairy on occasion, even though you know it doesn't make you feel your best. At least you will be able to make an educated decision. It is also possible that after being dairy-free for a while, your body will go back to tolerating small amounts of some dairy products.

Monday: _____

_____

_____

_____

_____

LESSON RECAP
Many adults lack the enzymes to efficiently digest dairy. The best way to learn what makes you feel your best is to experiment – even if you decide to consume dairy on occasion.

Tuesday: _____

_____

_____

_____

_____

Wednesday:_____

_____

_____

ACTION ITEM
Cut out all dairy products this week and monitor how you feel without them.

_____

Thursday: _____

_____

_____

_____

HEALTHY HABIT CHECKLIST

☐ Remember where you started & why
☐ Remember your goals
☐ Drink water
☐ Add in to crowd out
☐ Eat vegetables
☐ Eat healthy fats
☐ Chew your food
☐ Monitor cravings
☐ Bioindividuality
☐ Consider career
☐ New habits
☐ Probiotics
☐ Quiet connection
☐ Move your body
☐ Sugar
☐ Whole grains
☐ Sleep
☐ No processed food
☐ Home-cooked meals
☐ Gratitude
☐ Eating out
☐ Relationships
☐ Vitamin D
☐ Meat
☐ Dairy

Friday: _____

_____

_____

_____

_____

Saturday:_____

_____

_____

_____

Sunday:_____

_____

_____

_____

Weekly Summary: _____

_____

_____

_____

_____

_____

_____

WEEK TWENTY-SIX

"We don't experience natural environments enough to realize how restored they can make us feel."
~Florence Williams

When you are stressed, whether the cause is real or contrived, your body's stress hormones increase. One of the results of this reaction is that your body will hold onto stored fat, making it more difficult or impossible to lose weight regardless of your nutrition intake.

What is contrived stress? When you worry about being late for a meeting or getting your child to school, when you run from one thing to the next in a somewhat manic state, your body may perceive that you are under stress. Your nervous system does not know that your safety is not really in danger. It does what would be needed if you had been chased by a wild animal – it replenishes fat stores as if they had been used up and continues to store fat for future fight-or-flight responses.

Many of the habits throughout this book will help reduce your stress response. Staying hydrated, cultivating gratitude, meditating, eating nutritious food – all will play a role. Another practice that is shown to have a calming effect is to spend time in nature. A study in Japan tested people after a leisurely forest walk and after a walk in an urban setting. They found that compared to the urban walkers, the forest group had an average 12% reduction in cortisol levels (a stress hormone), a 7% reduction in sympathetic nervous activity (another stress marker), a 1.4% drop in blood pressure, a 6% drop in heart rate, and subjective reports of elevated mood and lower anxiety[1]. If you do not have time to get to a forest, spending time in a green space such as a park or a garden has been found to have a positive effect on one's health as well. This week, spend at least 10 minutes outside per day, not including time spent walking between your car and a building. You can sit, walk, or stand. Try to find a place without pavement.

---

[1] Florence Williams, *The Nature Fix* (New York: W.W. Norton, 2017), 23.

Monday: _____

_____

LESSON RECAP
Constant stress is
unhealthy, and yet
it is a state that
many people are in
on a regular basis
in our fast-paced,
guilt-ridden, busy
world. Getting
outside is one way
to reduce stress
hormones and
bring positive
physical and
mental changes.

Tuesday: _____

_____

_____

_____

_____

Wednesday:_____

_____

ACTION ITEM
Spend at least 10
minutes outside
each day this
week. Try to get
off pavement, or
at least be in a
garden or forest,
even if on
pavement. You can
walk, sit, or stand
– whatever suits
you. Throughout
the week, monitor
how it makes you
feel.

_____

_____

Thursday: _____

_____

_____

_____

_____

HEALTHY HABIT CHECKLIST

- ☐ Remember where you started & why
- ☐ Remember your goals
- ☐ Drink water
- ☐ Add in to crowd out
- ☐ Eat vegetables
- ☐ Eat healthy fats
- ☐ Chew your food
- ☐ Monitor cravings
- ☐ Bioindividuality
- ☐ Consider career
- ☐ New habits
- ☐ Probiotics
- ☐ Quiet connection
- ☐ Move your body
- ☐ Sugar
- ☐ Whole grains
- ☐ Sleep
- ☐ No processed food
- ☐ Home-cooked meals
- ☐ Gratitude
- ☐ Eating out
- ☐ Relationships
- ☐ Vitamin D
- ☐ Meat
- ☐ Dairy
- ☐ Get outside

Friday: _____

_____

_____

_____

_____

Saturday:_____

_____

_____

_____

_____

Sunday:_____

_____

_____

_____

_____

Weekly Summary: _____

_____

_____

_____

_____

_____

_____

_____

WEEK TWENTY-SEVEN

"There are plenty of obstacles in your path. Don't allow yourself to become one of them."
~Ralph Marston

Have you ever had a great date night with your significant other and then started an argument later in the evening? Have you received a great job offer and then spent your evening worried about something inconsequential?

This habit of getting in our own way is a phenomenon often referred to as self-sabotage. When something is going well in one area of our lives, we will often unconsciously do something either to harm that area of our lives, or to throw a wrench into a different area.

In his book, *The Big Leap,* Gay Hendricks refers to this as the Upper Limit Problem. He theorizes that we each have a set limit for how much good (wealth, health, success, etc.) we can take in our lives. When we get past that point of comfort, we do something to bring us back down within our comfort zone.

To get past this hurdle, we must first be aware of it. Then we must go about the work of convincing ourselves that we do deserve to expand that upper limit. Whatever abundance is coming to you (assuming it is sought and delivered in an ethical manner), it is something that you deserve to enjoy. Happiness is not part of a pie. Generally, your experience of abundance does not take away from anyone else. To the contrary, it is likely to spread rather than dwindle. Get comfortable with who you are now, as you are now. Enjoy your successes and your whole self. Then consider what you want for yourself, and continue to remind yourself that you deserve those things. If you recognize that you are about to self-sabotage, take a deep breath and reach out to someone if you can or find a way to break the cycle. If you realize it after the fact, take it as a learning experience and plan how to halt yourself next time.

LESSON RECAP
If you find yourself throwing a wrench into your life when things seem to be going well, you may be practicing self-sabotage. This may be because of a deep-seated belief that you do not deserve greater abundance. With time and keen awareness, you can teach yourself to allow greater abundance into your life.

ACTION ITEM
Can you think of a time that you practiced self-sabotage? Can you identify what was going on to cause it? This reflection may surprise you. Start trying to identify patterns, and then begin to change your behaviors and recognize that you deserve the abundance coming to you.

Monday: _____

_____

_____

_____

_____

Tuesday: _____

_____

_____

_____

_____

Wednesday:_____

_____

_____

_____

_____

Thursday: _____

_____

_____

_____

_____

**HEALTHY HABIT
CHECKLIST**
- □ Remember where you started & why
- □ Remember your goals
- □ Drink water
- □ Add in to crowd out
- □ Eat vegetables
- □ Eat healthy fats
- □ Chew your food
- □ Monitor cravings
- □ Bioindividuality
- □ Consider career
- □ New habits
- □ Probiotics
- □ Quiet connection
- □ Move your body
- □ Sugar
- □ Whole grains
- □ Sleep
- □ No processed food
- □ Home-cooked meals
- □ Gratitude
- □ Eating out
- □ Relationships
- □ Vitamin D
- □ Meat
- □ Dairy
- □ Get outside
- □ Self-sabotage

Friday: _____

_____

_____

_____

_____

Saturday:_____

_____

_____

_____

_____

Sunday:_____

_____

_____

_____

_____

Weekly Summary: _____

_____

_____

_____

_____

_____

_____

_____

WEEK TWENTY-EIGHT

TAKING CARE OF YOUR HOME ENVIRONMENT

"Outer Order. Inner Calm."
~Gretchen Rubin

Gretchen Rubin often says (and recently wrote a book by the same name): outer order, inner calm. In other words, when the environment around us is organized, we are more likely to feel calm and relaxed on the inside.

Many of us accumulate, accumulate, accumulate, without ever sending things OUT of the house.

Instead of organizing or discarding items piecemeal, organizer Marie Kondo suggests tackling entire categories at a time; and then keeping up as time goes on after the initial purge. For example, you could go through all linens, or all towels, or all jackets (if you do not want to do all clothes at once), or all the pens in your home. When you choose a type of object, she recommends that you gather all items together in one place, and then that you go through them one by one, hold the item, and decide whether to keep it or not by deciding whether it sparks joy in you. This will be more relevant for some than others. If nothing sparks joy, stick to the practical. Do you really need all of those t-shirts? Is it responsible to keep that paperwork?

Most of us have a pile of clothes that we hope to fit into again, someday. Instead of holding onto that hope, let them go. When you are a different size, you can enjoy getting clothes that fit will at that time.

There are many ways to donate items that someone else may want. That will be different for each region, but do some research ahead of time. It may be easier to get rid of items if you know that they will have a place to go.

WEEK TWENTY-EIGHT

LESSON RECAP
Clutter in your house can cause internal stress even if you do not recognize it. One way to organize is to go through categories of items all at once to decide what you really need around at this point in your life. If it rings true for you, keep only what sparks joy for you. Search for Marie Kondo for more information on this method.

ACTION ITEM Pick one category in your home or office to organize this week. Gather all like-items together and keep only what you need.

Monday: _____

_____

_____

_____

_____

Tuesday: _____

_____

_____

_____

_____

Wednesday:_____

_____

_____

_____

_____

Thursday: _____

_____

_____

_____

_____

Friday: _____

HEALTHY HABIT CHECKLIST

- ☐ Remember where you started & why
- ☐ Remember your goals
- ☐ Drink water
- ☐ Add in to crowd out
- ☐ Eat vegetables
- ☐ Eat healthy fats
- ☐ Chew your food
- ☐ Monitor cravings
- ☐ Bioindividuality
- ☐ Consider career
- ☐ New habits
- ☐ Probiotics
- ☐ Quiet connection
- ☐ Move your body
- ☐ Sugar
- ☐ Whole grains
- ☐ Sleep
- ☐ No processed food
- ☐ Home-cooked meals
- ☐ Gratitude
- ☐ Eating out
- ☐ Relationships
- ☐ Vitamin D
- ☐ Meat
- ☐ Dairy
- ☐ Get outside
- ☐ Self-sabotage
- ☐ Home environment

_____
_____
_____
_____

Saturday:_____

_____
_____
_____
_____

Sunday:_____

_____
_____
_____
_____

Weekly Summary: _____

_____
_____
_____
_____
_____
_____
_____
_____

WEEK TWENTY-NINE

THE 80/20 RULE

"Success doesn't come from what you do occasionally, it comes from what you do consistently."
~Marie Forleo

Being healthy for life means being flexible. Diets rarely work long-term because they are too strict and then the dieter rebels and 'eats all the things' until all of the lost weight (or even more) comes back. Food is much more than just the calories and nutrients. While eating a whole foods diet is the best way to eat most of the time, some foods hold deep traditional meaning far greater and more beneficial than any damage done from the calories and other additives.

One way to think about this is to eat those good, nourishing, whole foods roughly 80% of the time, leaving 20% for anything else. This could be weekly, or daily, or yearly. It will depend on your own eccentricities and it may take time to learn what works best for you. Hopefully it will take away any guilt from the occasional splurge or special occasion, without giving you an unlimited pass to eat unhealthy foods that will leave you feeling crummy.

As you begin to eat a cleaner diet, it may surprise you to learn that some of the crap foods you used to eat without noticing any change, now make you feel crummy. For that reason, and in the interest of your own health, most of these treats should be of high quality. Rather than a store-bought packaged muffin, choose a fresh muffin from a local bakery. Dark chocolate is better than milk chocolate. Homemade pizza is healthier than home delivery. What you choose to splurge on may change over time as your tastes change; for now, it may be the items that you are just not ready to give up even though you know they are not the best for you. That's okay, and you may be ready later to cut back or say goodbye.

Monday: _____
_____
_____
_____
_____

LESSON RECAP
To make healthy
eating a habit that
lasts for your
lifetime, it needs
to be flexible to fit
into whatever you
really care about,
and to allow the
occasional treat.
Eating well most of
the time is what
will matter in the
long term, not
what you do
occasionally. One
way to think about
this is to think
about eating well
80% of the time.

Tuesday: _____
_____
_____
_____
_____

Wednesday:_____
_____
_____
_____

ACTION ITEM
Reflect on your
thoughts on this
lesson. How can
you implement the
80/20 to make it
work for *you*?
Then put it into
action, modifying it
to your needs over
time.

Thursday: _____
_____
_____
_____

Friday: _____

HEALTHY HABIT CHECKLIST

□ Remember where you started & why
□ Remember your goals
□ Drink water
□ Add in to crowd out
□ Eat vegetables
□ Eat healthy fats
□ Chew your food
□ Monitor cravings
□ Bioindividuality
□ Consider career
□ New habits
□ Probiotics
□ Quiet connection
□ Move your body
□ Sugar
□ Whole grains
□ Sleep
□ No processed food
□ Home-cooked meals
□ Gratitude
□ Eating out
□ Relationships
□ Vitamin D
□ Meat
□ Dairy
□ Get outside
□ Self-sabotage
□ Home environment
□ The 80/20 rule

_____
_____
_____
_____

Saturday:_____

_____
_____
_____
_____

Sunday:_____

_____
_____
_____
_____

Weekly Summary: _____

_____
_____
_____
_____
_____
_____
_____
_____

WEEK THIRTY

"Think for yourself while being radically open-minded."
~Ray Dalio

Congratulations on completing this thirty-week healthy foundations program! Consistently moving forward through the lessons and making changes in how you think and live is no small feat.

Use this week to reflect on the changes you have made in the last 30 weeks and to decide what's next for you on your health journey. You will find questions to prompt your thinking on the following pages. Go back through the notes you have taken along the way, as well as your previous goals, to help you recall how far you have come. Keep your eye out for patterns as well to help you determine where to head next.

Complete another circle of life. Do so before revisiting the two previously-completed versions. Also revisit your measurements after these 30 weeks from page four, putting your current number next to your previous number and recording the date.

Whether we meet again or not, I wish you the very best on your health journey! May you feel happier and healthier each year that you continue living on this planet.

CIRCLE OF LIFE

Complete the circle of life one final time. Place a dot in the wedge for each category to indicate your level of satisfaction in that area. The center of the circle indicates zero satisfaction in that area; the outer edge indicates complete satisfaction in that area. Satisfaction means you do not feel there is room for improvement at this time in your life. Focus only on how you feel at this time. For example, education may not play a big role in your life right now, but if you are completely satisfied and do not wish to increase its role at this time, then you would put your dot near the outer edge of the circle. When you are done, connect the dots.

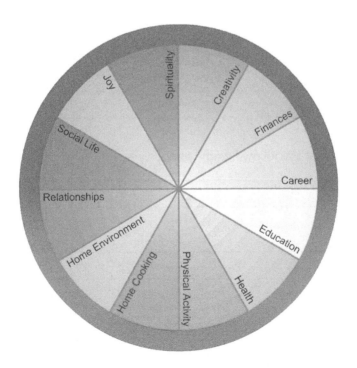

REFLECTION

Since starting this program I have made the following changes:

I am really proud of myself for: _____

_____

I learned that the following habits/foods, etc. make me feel great:

_____

I observe the following patterns in my behavior: _____

_____

The single biggest thing I can do now for my health is: _____

_____

My biggest struggle is: _____

_____

My top goals for the following time periods are:
30 days_____

_____

60 days_____

_____

6 months_____

_____

1 year _____

_____

Monday: _____

_____

_____

_____

_____

LESSON RECAP
Congratulations on making small consistent change for the last 30 weeks! Reflect on your journey, take some time to be proud of yourself, and if you got behind, no worries: make a plan to catch up.

Tuesday: _____

_____

_____

_____

_____

Wednesday:_____

_____

ACTION ITEM
Complete the Circle of Life and then compare to the two you did previously. Look at your goals from the beginning your notes throughout this book. Take time with the reflection questions to move your forward.

_____

_____

_____

Thursday: _____

_____

_____

_____

_____

HEALTHY HABIT CHECKLIST

- ☐ Remember where you started & why
- ☐ Remember your goals
- ☐ Drink water
- ☐ Add in to crowd out
- ☐ Eat vegetables
- ☐ Eat healthy fats
- ☐ Chew your food
- ☐ Monitor cravings
- ☐ Bioindividuality
- ☐ Consider career
- ☐ New habits
- ☐ Probiotics
- ☐ Quiet connection
- ☐ Move your body
- ☐ Sugar
- ☐ Whole grains
- ☐ Sleep
- ☐ No processed food
- ☐ Home-cooked meals
- ☐ Gratitude
- ☐ Eating out
- ☐ Relationships
- ☐ Vitamin D
- ☐ Meat
- ☐ Dairy
- ☐ Get outside
- ☐ Self-sabotage
- ☐ Home environment
- ☐ The 80/20 rule
- ☐ Reflection & what's next

Friday: _____

_____

_____

_____

_____

Saturday: _____

_____

_____

_____

_____

Sunday: _____

_____

_____

Weekly Summary: _____

_____

_____

_____

_____

_____

_____

BONUS – FOR TRAVEL

"Travel and change of place impart new vigour to the mind."
~Seneca

It is easiest to achieve health at home by creating routines. A few weeks ago, we covered the importance of meal preparation, including a tip to buy essentially the same things over and over so that you do not have to recreate a brand-new shopping list each week. Travel, whether for work or for play, can upend all of that. Cooking may not be an option, and it may be more difficult to find certain foods. If travel is stressful for you, it might also set off emotional eating.

Yet, as with most things, a little bit of planning ahead can go a long way. When possible, choose a room with a kitchen or as close as you can get to it. A mini-fridge and a microwave allow for good, healthy meal preparation. Once settled, take a trip to the store to stock up on vegetables and fruits for snacks or meals. If you will have the opportunity to eat in your room, consider simple options such as salad (buy lettuce and dressing; you could also buy toppings from a salad bar if available), canned soup that can be heated up, or a sweet potato, which you can cook in the microwave.

Make sure you always have healthy snacks such as nuts, fruit, vegetables, hard-boiled eggs, or some kind of nut or date bar with whole food ingredients. When you do eat out, use tips from the eating out lesson.

Occasionally enjoy good, local food, regardless of ingredients. It's a benefit of travel. Don't worry and don't regret it.

Finally, make sure to incorporate movement while away from home. Walking can be a great way of exploring a new place (if it's safe; use a treadmill if not). Exercise will assist you in your effort to eat better and keep you feeling better overall.

LESSON RECAP
Leaving home for work or vacation does not have to mean eating unhealthy foods that will leave you feeling crummy. You may be eating different food, but with some forethought you can make great choices while away.

ACTION ITEM
Focus on eating so you feel your best. Make good choices most of the time, and enjoy regional specialties occasionally as well.

Monday: _____

_____

_____

_____

_____

Tuesday: _____

_____

_____

_____

_____

Wednesday:_____

_____

_____

_____

_____

Thursday: _____

_____

_____

_____

_____

HEALTHY HABIT CHECKLIST

☐ Remember where you started & why
☐ Remember your goals
☐ Drink water
☐ Add in to crowd out
☐ Eat vegetables
☐ Eat healthy fats
☐ Chew your food
☐ Monitor cravings
☐ Bioindividuality
☐ Consider career
☐ New habits
☐ Probiotics
☐ Quiet connection
☐ Move your body
☐ Sugar
☐ Whole grains
☐ Sleep
☐ No processed food
☐ Home-cooked meals
☐ Gratitude
☐ Eating out
☐ Relationships
☐ Vitamin D
☐ Meat
☐ Dairy
☐ Get outside
☐ Self-sabotage
☐ Home environment
☐ The 80/20 rule
☐ Reflection & what's next
☐ Bonus: Travel

Friday: _____

_____

_____

_____

_____

Saturday:_____

_____

_____

_____

_____

Sunday:_____

_____

_____

_____

_____

Weekly Summary: _____

_____

_____

_____

_____

_____

_____

_____

BONUS – LIFE HAPPENS

WHEN LIFE GETS IN THE WAY

"The whole future lies in uncertainty: Live immediately."
~Seneca

This book is designed for you to focus on one new habit every week for over a half a year of your life! While this time is short as a percentage of the many years you will hopefully be alive, it is nonetheless a significant period of time. During this period, it is likely that you will face hardships and/or disruptions to your schedule. You will experience weeks when you feel great and are motivated to keep up on your new healthy habits. Other weeks, you may want to throw this book in the fire and stop thinking about anything new.

When events that disrupt your life for better and for worse arise, what do you do? Instead of abandoning this book, turn to this section for thoughts about how to move forward. Consider these suggestions:

- Remember that your action item each week is supposed to be small and easy. Pick an action item in this current week's lesson that sounds absurdly easy and *only* focus on that during the week. There are reminders each week about what you have already covered, but now is not the time to do everything. In this moment, focus as small as you can, but still focus and move forward.
- Alternatively, maybe you need to choose your own focus for the week. Take a week off of the book's topics and decide what you need the most. Commit to that focus all week.
- If you do end up putting this book aside for a period of time, when you are ready, pick right back up where you left off and keep moving forward.
- If you find yourself gravitating towards unhealthy habits, try to be observant rather than judgmental. Why are you doing it? What emotions are you seeking? Are you actually finding comfort? Journal or talk with a friend to find the why, rather than being upset with yourself. Digging deep on your 'why' will provide insight on the trigger, and from there you can decide what you want to do next.